HOW TO SOOTHE THE BURN

A GUIDE TO MANAGING HEARTBURN DURING PREGNANCY

Expert Advice and Natural Remedies for a Comfortable Pregnancy Journey

By

Lena M. Hughes

Table of Contents

Introduction...v

Welcome to the Journey of Pregnancy........... vii

Chapter 1 1

Understanding Heartburn during Pregnancy.....1

What causes heartburn during pregnancy?........3

What exactly is acid reflux in pregnancy? 6

Chapter 2 8

Heartburn Symptoms and Diagnosis.................8

Heartburn Signs and Symptoms 8

Heartburn Diagnose 10

Chapter 3 12

Natural Heartburn Treatments during

Pregnancy 12

Nutritional Modifications 15

Changes in Lifestyle 17

Natural Treatments 19

When should I contact my doctor regarding

heartburn during pregnancy? 21

Chapter 4 23

Medicines for Heartburn during Pregnancy 23

Avoiding Heartburn during Pregnancy 29

Foods that will not give you heartburn............34

Healthy Habits for a Relaxed Pregnancy 37

Conclusion 41

Heartburn-Friendly Foods and Snacks............43

Introduction

Pregnancy is a beautiful time in a woman's life but it also has difficulties. Heartburn is one of the most prevalent complaints among pregnant women. Heartburn can be uncomfortable and painful during pregnancy, making it difficult to enjoy this beautiful time.

In this book, How to Soothe the Burn: A Guide to Managing Heartburn during Pregnancy, we will look at the origins, symptoms, and natural therapies for heartburn during pregnancy. We will discuss the safe drugs during pregnancy and offer heartburn prevention methods.

Being a mother, I realize how tough it can be to handle pregnancy heartburn. That is why I wrote this book to assist expectant mothers in navigating this frequent difficulty with confidence and ease. Whether you suffer from mild or severe heartburn, this book will provide you with the knowledge and techniques to manage it properly and enjoy your pregnancy experience fully.

So, let's dig in and discover the realm of heartburn in pregnancy together.

Welcome to the Journey of Pregnancy

Pregnancy is a special and precious time in a woman's life. It is a period of growth, change, and transition, both physically and mentally. The minute you find out you're pregnant, you go on a path of self-discovery and exploration. You will learn about your body, baby, and yourself in ways you never imagined.

This trip will be full of ups and downs, but it's vital to remember that every experience is genuine and natural. You will likely experience various emotions, from excitement and delight to dread and uncertainty. It's crucial to take care of yourself during this time, both physically and mentally.

Pregnancy can also come with obstacles, including morning sickness, exhaustion, heartburn, and potential concerns such as gestational diabetes and preeclampsia.

Nonetheless, with adequate care and attention, most women can have healthy pregnancies and give birth to healthy kids.

This book focuses on one of pregnancy's significant difficulties: heartburn. I will give you information, strategies, and resources to help you manage this disease and enjoy your pregnancy adventure to the utmost.

Pregnancy is a journey, and no two trips are the same. Enjoy the experience, seek help and counsel as required, and care for yourself and your growing kid.

Chapter 1
Understanding Heartburn during Pregnancy

Heartburn is a frequent ailment that affects many pregnant women. It is a burning feeling in the chest and throat and might be accompanied by a sour taste in the mouth. Heartburn is produced by stomach acid refluxing into the oesophagus, the tube connecting the mouth to the stomach.

Throughout pregnancy, the risk of heartburn increases due to hormonal and physical changes in the body. The hormone progesterone, generated at higher levels during pregnancy, can cause the valve between the stomach and oesophagus to relax, allowing stomach acid to flow back into the oesophagus more easily. The developing uterus can also pressure the stomach, sending stomach acid into the oesophagus.

Heartburn during pregnancy can be

uncomfortable and interfere with daily activities, but it is usually not a cause for concern. However, if you feel severe or persistent heartburn, it is crucial to contact your healthcare physician since this could indicate a more severe illness.

In the following sections of this book, we will examine the causes, symptoms, and natural cures for heartburn during pregnancy and suggestions for preventing and treating this problem.

What causes heartburn during pregnancy?

Heartburn is when you experience a burning sensation in your chest. The painful sensation can migrate up your throat. You may also feel a bitter or sour taste in the back of your throat.

Despite it being termed "heartburn," it's unrelated to your heart. It happens because of acid reflux when stomach acid flows from your stomach up to your oesophagus. The oesophagus is the tube that delivers food, fluids and saliva to your stomach.

Heartburn is a frequent sensation experienced by pregnant women. Hormonal changes and changes in body form can cause heartburn.

- **Hormonal Shifts**

Heartburn can be exacerbated by hormonal changes during pregnancy. The hormone progesterone generated more significantly during pregnancy, can relax the valve between the stomach and the oesophagus, allowing stomach acid to flow freely into the oesophagus. This valve relaxation is required to accommodate the expanding uterus and developing fetus.

Besides relaxing the valve, Progesterone inhibits digestion, which can lead to an accumulation of stomach acid. As a result, pregnant women may experience more frequent and severe heartburn attacks.

While hormonal changes cannot be avoided during pregnancy, there are things you may take to manage heartburn symptoms.

• Expanding Uterus and Digestive System Stress

During pregnancy, the uterus expands, putting pressure on the digestive system, including the stomach and intestines. This pressure can force stomach acid back into the oesophagus, resulting in heartburn.

Pressure on the stomach can also impact digestion, causing food to move more slowly through the digestive tract. Slower digestion might result in an accumulation of stomach acid, exacerbating heartburn symptoms.

The developing uterus can strain the diaphragm, the muscle that separates the chest and abdominal chambers, and the digestive system. This can make the diaphragm work harder, causing breathing difficulty and worsening heartburn sensations.

• Lower oesophagal sphincter relaxation

The pregnancy hormone progesterone can cause the lower oesophagal sphincter to relax. Stomach acid can flow up into the oesophagus when it relaxes.

What exactly is acid reflux in pregnancy?

The terms "heartburn" and "acid reflux" are interchangeable. However, their definitions differ:

• Acid reflux is caused by the LES not constricting properly. This allows gastric acid to pass from the stomach to the oesophagus. (GERD, or gastroesophageal reflux disease, is a severe form of acid reflux.)

• Heartburn, or a burning sensation in your chest, is a symptom of acid reflux.

Due to shifting hormone levels and the baby's growth, women may feel acid reflux and heartburn throughout pregnancy.

Is heartburn common during pregnancy?

Over half of the pregnant women experience severe heartburn throughout the third trimester.

Chapter 2

Heartburn Symptoms and Diagnosis

Heartburn is a frequent pregnant symptom described as a burning sensation in the chest or throat. A sour feeling in the mouth or regurgitation of food or liquid might also accompany it. Heartburn symptoms usually appear after eating or lying down and might linger for several hours.

You must contact your healthcare professional immediately if you have any of these signs. They can do tests to establish the underlying cause of your symptoms and propose the best course of action.

Heartburn Signs and Symptoms

Heartburn is a typical pregnancy symptom that can be uncomfortable and disruptive. Some signs and symptoms of heartburn during pregnancy include:

1. A burning sensation in the chest or throat following a meal.

2. A bitter aftertaste in the mouth or throat.

3. Upper abdominal pain or discomfort

4. Trouble swallowing

5. Feeling full or bloated

6. Vomiting or nausea

7. Burping or belching

8. Bring up food

These symptoms are caused by stomach acid backing up into the oesophagus and usually, appear after eating or lying down. Heartburn symptoms can be minor to severe, and they can last for several hours.

While heartburn is usually not a cause for concern during pregnancy, it is vital to be aware of the signs and symptoms of more serious illnesses, such as preeclampsia or HELLP syndrome. These disorders can include severe or chronic heartburn, vomiting blood or material resembling coffee grounds, chest pain or pressure, shortness of breath, and swelling in the hands, feet, or face.

If you have any of these symptoms, you must contact your healthcare professional immediately. They can do tests to establish the underlying cause of your symptoms and propose the best course of action. In the following sections of this book, we will address natural therapies, drugs, and lifestyle changes that can help relieve heartburn during pregnancy.

Heartburn Diagnose

Heartburn during pregnancy is usually diagnosed based on the symptoms and medical history of the woman. Your doctor will most likely inquire about the frequency and intensity of your heartburn symptoms and any other symptoms you may be experiencing.

In rare situations, your doctor may recommend additional testing to rule out other disorders causing your symptoms. Upper endoscopy, which employs a small camera to examine the lining of the oesophagus, stomach, and small intestine, is one of these examinations. Your healthcare professional may also perform a pH monitoring test to assess the acid in your oesophagus over 24 hours.

Heartburn during pregnancy is usually not a cause for concern and can often be treated with lifestyle changes and over-the-counter drugs.

However, suppose your symptoms are severe or persistent or accompanied by other painful symptoms, such as trouble swallowing or vomiting blood. In that case, you should contact your healthcare professional immediately.

Chapter 3

Natural Heartburn Treatments during Pregnancy

Heartburn can be uncomfortable and irritating during pregnancy, but some natural therapies can help ease symptoms. You can try the following natural remedies:

1. Eat smaller, more frequent meals: Eat several small meals throughout the day instead of three large ones. This can help lower the acid in your stomach and avoid heartburn.

2. Avoid trigger foods: Some foods, such as spicy or fatty foods, citrus fruits, chocolate, and coffee, can cause heartburn. Try to avoid or limit your consumption of these items to alleviate your symptoms.

3. Drinking enough water can help dilute stomach acid and lessen the risk of heartburn. Try to consume 8-10 glasses of water every day.

4. **Elevate your head when sleeping:** Although bedtime snacking and midday naps are difficult to avoid during pregnancy, reclining down after eating might cause heartburn. Lying down can increase stomach pressure, which can cause stomach acid to rise. You can prevent a sleepless night of heartburn by eating and digesting early in the evening.

Avoid lying down flat to help prevent mild heartburn. If you must lie down after eating, keep your head slightly elevated. This can help you avoid exerting too much pressure on your stomach, which could allow acid to escape.

Use a foam wedge or block to raise yourself into an elevated position at night to help reduce heartburn.

According to research, elevating the head of the bed can help alleviate acid reflux symptoms.

Remember that lifting your head is not a cure

for heartburn but a temporary solution.

This simple modification may not help if other pregnant factors, such as hormone changes, are causing your heartburn.

4. Dress comfortably: Tight clothing might put a strain on your abdomen and raise your risk of heartburn. To alleviate your symptoms, dress comfortably.

5. Use relaxation techniques: Because stress increases your risk of heartburn, it's critical to use forms of therapy such as breathing exercises, meditation, or yoga.

6. Try sleeping on your left side. Because your stomach is on the left, acids are more difficult to enter the oesophagus at this angle.

7. Chew on some gum. This produces more saliva containing bicarbonate, which, when ingested, neutralizes the acid in the oesophagus.

8. Use ginger: Ginger has anti-inflammatory

qualities that can assist with nausea and heartburn. To alleviate your symptoms, try drinking ginger tea or taking ginger pills.

While these natural solutions can assist with heartburn during pregnancy, you must consult your doctor before beginning any new treatment regimen. They can make personalized recommendations based on your medical history and current health situation.

Nutritional Modifications

Heartburn during pregnancy can be effectively managed with dietary adjustments. These are some nutritional modifications you can try:

1. **Eat slowly and thoroughly:** Eating too fast might lead to swallowing air, which can increase heartburn. Take your time when eating, and chew your food thoroughly.

2. **Avoid eating huge meals:** Eating large

meals might strain your stomach and increase your chances of experiencing heartburn. Eat smaller, more regular meals all day instead.

3. Avoid trigger foods: Some foods, such as spicy or fatty foods, citrus fruits, chocolate, and coffee, can cause heartburn. Try to avoid or limit your consumption of these items to alleviate your symptoms.

4. Eat low-fat foods: High-fat foods might slow digestion, increasing your risk of heartburn. Choose low-fat foods like lean proteins, fruits, vegetables, and whole grains instead.

5. Maintain an upright posture after eating: Laying down increases your heartburn risk. Instead, remain upright for at least 30 minutes after eating to allow food to digest properly.

6. Drinking enough water can help dilute stomach acid and lessen the risk of heartburn. Try to consume 8-10 glasses of water every day.

7. Drink in between meals, not with them.

8. Avoid eating before bed: Eating before bed can raise your risk of heartburn. Avoid eating for at least 2-3 hours before bedtime.

In addition to these dietary modifications, it is critical to maintain a healthy weight and avoid smoking, both of which can contribute to heartburn. If you need help making nutritional adjustments independently, consult a certified dietitian who can provide individualized suggestions based on your unique needs and preferences.

Changes in Lifestyle

In addition to nutritional changes, several lifestyle changes can help manage heartburn during pregnancy. These are some lifestyle changes you can try:

1. Avoid lying down after meals: Lying down after eating increases your chances of experiencing heartburn. Instead, remain upright for at least 30 minutes after eating to allow food to digest properly.

2. Dress comfortably: Tight clothing can pressure your abdomen and increase your risk of heartburn. To alleviate your symptoms, dress comfortably.

3. Sleep with your head elevated: Sleeping with your head promoted can help prevent stomach acid from flowing back into your oesophagus. While sleeping, use pillows to prop up your head and upper body.

4. Use stress-reduction techniques: Because stress increases your risk of heartburn, it's critical to use techniques such as deep breathing, meditation, or yoga.

5. Regular exercise can help improve digestion

and lower your risk of heartburn. Consult your doctor about safe exercise options during pregnancy.

6. Avoid smoking: Smoking increases your risk of heartburn by relaxing the muscle that separates the stomach and the oesophagus, allowing stomach acid to seep back into the oesophagus.

7. Maintain a healthy weight: Excess weight can put a strain on your abdomen and increase your chances of experiencing heartburn. Discuss appropriate weight control measures with your healthcare professional throughout pregnancy.

Natural Treatments

While herbal remedies are a popular option for treating heartburn during pregnancy, it is critical to consult your healthcare professional before attempting new herbal remedies. Certain herbs can be hazardous during pregnancy, so make sure any herbal cures you're contemplating are healthy for you and your baby.

These are some herbal remedies that may help with heartburn during pregnancy:

1. Ginger: Ginger has anti-inflammatory qualities that can help reduce oesophagal and stomach inflammation. Try drinking ginger tea or incorporating raw ginger into your meals.

2. Peppermint: Peppermint soothes heartburn and has a relaxing effect on the stomach. Consider drinking peppermint tea or chewing on peppermint leaves.

3. Licorice: Licorice has natural stomach-soothing effects and can help reduce oesophagal inflammation. Nevertheless, deglycyrrhizinated liquorice (DGL) is preferred because ordinary liquorice can raise blood pressure and create other harmful side effects.

4.   **Chamomile:**   Chamomile   is   anti-inflammatory and can help reduce oesophagal and stomach discomfort. Drink chamomile tea before or after meals.

5. **Slippery elm:** Slippery elm relaxes the stomach and can help reduce oesophagal irritation. It is offered as a supplement or as a tea.

When should I contact my doctor regarding heartburn during pregnancy?

If your heartburn persists, consult your healthcare physician. They can advise you on which medications are safe to use while pregnant.

You should also contact your doctor if you:

• have nighttime heartburn.

• have difficulty swallowing.

• spit blood.

• have black poop.

• are losing weight.

Heartburn symptoms can be identical to those of a heart attack. If you've never had heartburn before and are experiencing chest symptoms, contact your provider or visit the local emergency room.

Chapter 4
Medicines for Heartburn during Pregnancy

Many pregnant women experience heartburn, often known as acid indigestion or acid reflux. This condition is usually not dangerous, but it can be highly uncomfortable. Fortunately, the majority of instances may be safely treated with over-the-counter medications, as well as simple dietary and lifestyle adjustments.

Many women find that eating small, frequent meals and avoiding spicy or acidic foods helps them feel better. Several prescription and over-the-counter heartburn treatments are considered safe throughout pregnancy for people who require further assistance.

Here are some recommendations to help you understand which heartburn medications are safe while pregnant. *(As with any drug, consult your*

healthcare professional before using them.)

While natural therapies and lifestyle changes can help manage heartburn during pregnancy, medication may be required in certain circumstances to relieve symptoms. However, consult your healthcare professional before taking any medications because some drugs might be dangerous during pregnancy.

Antacids

Most over-the-counter antacids, including calcium carbonate (Tums), are safe to take while pregnant.

Antacids are commonly available in chewable tablets containing magnesium, aluminium, or calcium salts that help neutralize stomach acid and prevent a burning feeling.

If you frequently get heartburn after meals or before bed, taking an antacid with food or before bed can help temporarily ease heartburn.

Before taking an over-the-counter antacid, consult with your doctor. They can advise you on a suitable dosage and an antacid that is safe to use during pregnancy.

For example, sodium bicarbonate antacids (such as Alka-Seltzer) are not regarded safe for pregnancy since they can induce oedema and health concerns associated with the acid balance of your blood.

Because of non-pregnancy-safe components such as salicylates, antacids such as bismuth subsalicylate (Pepto Bismol) are also unsafe to ingest during pregnancy.

Unless you take exceptionally high dosages of a pregnancy-safe antacid, significant problems while pregnant are unusual.

Nevertheless, antacids can interfere with iron and folic acid absorption and should not be combined with other drugs or supplements, especially if you have a vitamin shortage. Antacids can also induce the following adverse effects:

- Diarrhea

- Constipation

- Headache

- Abdominal pain

A healthcare physician may recommend taking alginates along with antacids for further heartburn relief. Alginates are drugs that form a gel layer on top of your stomach acid, forming a barrier that keeps stomach acid from escaping.

H2 Blockers

If antacids and preventative measures do not relieve your heartburn, a more potent medicine, such as an H2 blocker, may be the next step.

These prescription or over-the-counter (OTC)

drugs, often known as H2 receptor blockers or H2 receptor antagonists (H2RAs), help restrict stomach acid production and cure heartburn.

H2RAs are the most commonly used medicine to manage acid reflux during pregnancy, after antacids. H2 blockers, such as famotidine (Pepcid), are considered safe during pregnancy. The blockers, however, are only approved by the US Food and Drug Administration as a short-term treatment for moderate heartburn or indigestion.

Before using any OTC medicine, consult with your doctor about which H2 blocker may alleviate your heartburn symptoms. They may propose an OTC alternative or prescription you an H2 blocker.

H2 blockers are unlikely to cause side effects but may cause diarrhoea, constipation, headaches, drowsiness, and abdominal discomfort. They may also interfere with some drugs, including theophylline, specific SSRIs, and warfarin. Proton

Pump Inhibitors

Proton pump inhibitors (PPIs) are a class of prescription and over-the-counter drugs, such as lansoprazole (Prevacid) that assist in reducing stomach acid production for heartburn relief.

These drugs are more potent than H2 blockers but also increase your chances of developing infections and bacterial overgrowth. Individuals should only use PPIs if they have acid reflux complications or other treatment options have failed.

While PPIs are excellent at reducing stomach acid, which can cause heartburn, they can be slow to function, causing relief to be delayed.

Most PPIs are safe for pregnant women. Omeprazole is an exception (Prilosec). Omeprazole has been demonstrated in animal tests to be harmful to a developing fetus, and healthcare specialists do not believe it is safe for human pregnancy.

While the risk of adverse effects is low when using PPIs for short periods and at moderate doses, some of the adverse effects of taking PPIs may include headache, dizziness, abdominal pain, diarrhoea, back pain, and upper respiratory infections.

Consult a healthcare physician to determine which PPI is best for you.

Avoiding Heartburn during Pregnancy

Nine heartburn home remedies

If you want to avoid acid reflux or get rid of heartburn quickly, here are nine techniques to alleviate and maybe eliminate your symptoms:

1. Maintain a food diary and avoid trigger foods.

As previously stated, certain meals and beverages can cause acid reflux and heartburn. Keeping a food and symptom journal will help you discover the items most likely to cause you problems. Once you've identified them, avoid them as much as possible.

2. Refrain from overeating or eating too rapidly.

When it comes to preventing heartburn, controlling portion amounts at meals can help. A large part of food in your stomach may strain the valve that keeps stomach acid out of your oesophagus, increasing the likelihood of acid reflux and heartburn. If you suffer from heartburn, try eating smaller meals more frequently. Eating fast can also cause heartburn, so take your time, chew your food, and sip your beverages.

3. Avoid eating late at night, snacking before bed, and eating before exercising.

Lying down with a full stomach might cause

acid reflux and worsen heartburn symptoms. Avoid eating within 3 hours of going to bed to give your stomach enough time to empty. You should also rest for at least two hours before exercising.

4. Consume alkaline foods such as ripe bananas.

A banana's high potassium content makes it an alkaline food. According to the Academy of Nutrition and Dietetics, this may assist in balancing the stomach acid that is irritating your oesophagus.

Nevertheless, there is one caveat: Unripe bananas are lower in alkalinity, contain more starch, and may cause acid reflux in some persons. Therefore make sure you select a ripe banana.

Melons, cauliflower, fennel, and nuts are some alkaline foods that may aid with heartburn.

5. Dress in loose-fitting attire.

Tight-fitting belts and garments that pinch your stomach may contribute to your heartburn problems.

6. Change your sleeping position

Sleeping with your head and chest higher than your feet can help prevent and relieve acid reflux and heartburn. This can be accomplished by placing a foam wedge under the mattress or lifting bedposts with wood blocks. Be wary of piling pillows, which are rarely helpful and may aggravate your symptoms. Sleeping on your left side is also known to promote digestion and may help to prevent stomach acid reflux.

7. If you are overweight, make efforts to decrease weight.

Heavy weight strains your stomach, increasing your chances of acid reflux and heartburn. The first two steps to maintaining a healthy weight and decreasing extra weight are eating a well-balanced diet and doing 150 minutes of physical exercise per week.

8. If you smoke, you should quit.

Smoking decreases the quantity of saliva produced and affects the efficacy of the valve that prevents stomach acid from entering the oesophagus, both of which increase the likelihood of heartburn. Stopping smoking can lower the intensity and frequency of acid reflux and, in some circumstances, remove it entirely.

9. Minimize stress. Prolonged stress physically impacts your body, delaying digestion and increasing pain sensitivity. The longer food remains in your stomach; the more likely stomach acid may reflux. Also, having an enhanced sensitivity to pain might intensify the burning agony of heartburn. Taking action to lessen stress may aid in the prevention or relief of acid reflux and heartburn.

Foods that will not give you heartburn

Some meals are beneficial in relieving or assisting with heartburn symptoms.

1. Milk

It has been shown that drinking milk can help ease the discomfort caused by heartburn. Because milk has an alkaline content, it helps to form a thin barrier that coats the stomach and can reduce inflammation.

Skimmed or semi-skimmed milk is preferred because high-fat milk sources might aggravate heartburn.

Pregnant women need 700mg of calcium daily, and 100 ml of milk has 120mg. As a result, milk is an excellent source of calcium and should be included in your diet to maintain bone health. Milk can be added to cereal, used as an ingredient in cooking, or used as the primary liquid foundation for a smoothie or hot drink.

2. Teas made from herbs

Home cures for heartburn include herbal teas such as ginger, fennel, and peppermint. While there is little scientific proof that herbal teas can prevent heartburn, pregnant women have reported good outcomes in reducing symptoms. As a result, you could consume herbal teas in between meals as a healthy source of water, which may help avoid or ease heartburn symptoms.

3. Foods fermented

Sauerkraut, kefir, and tempeh are examples of fermented foods high in probiotics. Probiotics are good for our digestion and gut microbiome, as well as encouraging the secretion of digestive juices, which can aid in the regularity of our digestive systems. In some circumstances, this helps prevent problems like indigestion and heartburn. Include 1-2 servings of these foods in your daily diet.

4. Yoghurt

Yoghurt, like milk, can assist in reducing the irritation produced by heartburn. It is a probiotic and alkaline source that can neutralise stomach acid.

Yoghurt is another source of calcium and protein that can help you reach your nutritional needs. Selecting plain, low-fat yoghurt is usually the best option for heartburn treatment, so consider incorporating it into a snack or using it as a savoury dip at a meal to help reduce the risk of heartburn.

5. Bananas and melons

Melons and bananas are less acidic than most fruits. As a result, they are ideal options for getting one of your five a day and meeting your fibre needs without causing heartburn symptoms. Both fruits can be eaten as a snack with yoghurt or mixed into your morning cereal or oatmeal.

6. Whole grains

Fibre-rich whole grains include brown rice, pasta, whole-grain bread, and oats. In some situations, fibre can assist in speeding up the digestion of food via the stomach, keeping food from being in the stomach for longer than necessary, and limiting the quantity of acid produced. As a result, the likelihood of acid reflux may be reduced.

To add whole grains into your diet, replace white bread with brown or rye bread for toast or a sandwich at lunch. You could also cook an oat-based breakfast, such as porridge or a flapjack bar.

Healthy Habits for a Relaxed Pregnancy

You must first take care of yourself and your unborn child before you can care for your new baby. There is a lot of guidance available.

1. Consume a prenatal vitamin.

2. Work out regularly

3. Create a birth plan

4. Educate yourself.

5. Alter your chores (avoid harsh or toxic cleaners and heavy lifting)

6. Monitor your weight growth (average weight gain is 25-35 pounds)

7. Purchase comfy shoes

8. Consume folate-rich meals (lentils, asparagus, oranges, fortified cereals)

9. Consume calcium-rich meals (dairy, canned fish, soy)

10. Consume more fish (except those high in mercury)

11. Consume fibre-rich meals

12. Avoid eating soft cheeses (unpasteurized styles like Brie and feta may contain bacteria that can cause fever, miscarriage or pregnancy

complications)

13. Consume your vegetables

14. Have five to six well-balanced meals per day.

15. But do not overeat. You require 300-500 more calories every day. Maintain a food journal.

Restrict your caffeine intake.

17. Consume plenty of water (six 8-ounce glasses of water per day)

18. Avoid consuming alcoholic beverages.

19. Wear sunscreen.

20. Fly wisely (avoid air travel if possible early and late in pregnancy)

21. Avoid replacing kitty litter (to reduce the risk of toxoplasmosis)

22. Give in to urges on occasion

23. Know when to contact your doctor if you have any concerns.

24. Quit smoking and avoid secondhand smoke.

25. Get enough rest.

26. Wear your seatbelt.

27. Consult a doctor before using over-the-counter drugs or natural therapies.

28. See your dentist

29. Attend a pregnancy class

30. Babysit a friend's child to gain practical experience.

31. Visit birthing facilities

32. Use relaxation practices daily (yoga, stretching, deep breathing, massage)

33. Avoid overmedicating

34. Work out, but not excessively.

35. Stretch before bed to avoid leg cramps.

36. Before the baby arrives, take a picture of yourself.

Conclusion

Finally, heartburn is a common and often unpleasant symptom of pregnancy. While it can be challenging to prevent and manage, there are numerous ways you can employ to reduce symptoms and enhance your overall comfort. Multiple therapeutic options for treating heartburn during pregnancy include food and lifestyle changes to natural therapies and pharmaceuticals. Consult your healthcare professional for advice and support if you have severe or chronic heartburn. You may have a safe and comfortable pregnancy with the proper care and attention.

Finally, some words of encouragement and support:

As you go through the stages of pregnancy, keep in mind that each woman's experience is unique. Some people get heartburn, whereas others don't. Whatever obstacles you confront, it's critical to prioritize self-care and seek the help you need to manage your symptoms and stay well. Remember that your healthcare practitioner is always there to answer your questions and provide direction, and numerous resources assist you during this exciting and changing time. Above all, believe in your strength and perseverance, and know that you can handle anything that comes your way.

Heartburn-Friendly Foods and Snacks

• Chicken and Vegetable Stir Fry: Cut boneless, skinless chicken breast into bite-sized pieces and stir fry with garlic, ginger, and your choice of vegetables on a nonstick skillet (e.g. broccoli, carrots, bell peppers). Over brown rice or quinoa, serve.

• Sweet Potato and Black Bean Tacos: Toss cubed sweet potato with black beans, sliced onion, diced tomato, and taco seasoning after roasting until cooked. Serve with avocado and salsa in soft tortillas.

• Greek Yogurt Parfait: In a tall glass, layer Greek yoghurt, sliced banana, and granola. Pour honey over the top and sprinkle with cinnamon.

• Fish with Roasted Vegetables: Season salmon fillets with salt, pepper, and lemon juice, then bake for 15-20 minutes at 400 degrees. Serve alongside roasted veggies like asparagus, zucchini, and bell peppers.

• In a blender, combine frozen mixed berries, almond milk, and banana until smooth. Top with sliced banana, almonds, and chia seeds in a bowl.

These recipes are a starting point; you can change them to suit your unique tastes and dietary requirements. It's critical to avoid heartburn trigger foods like citrus, tomatoes, spicy foods, and caffeine while cooking for heartburn during pregnancy. Instead, concentrate on lean meats, healthy grains, and nutrient-dense fruits and vegetables.